Keto Diet Recipes in 30 Minutes

Gorgeous Ketogenic Diet Recipes, Super Easy to Prepare for Busy People. This Guide Will Help You Lose Weight Faster

Sarah Vellar

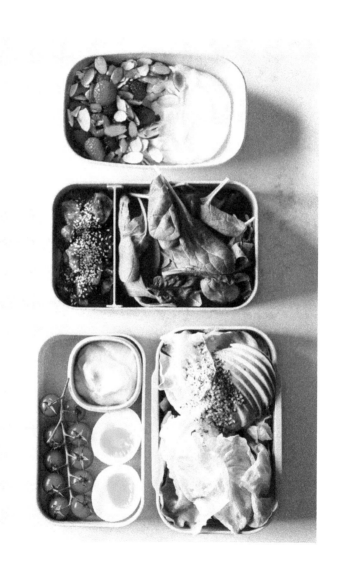

Table of Contents

INTRODUCTION

So the Ketogenic Diet is all about reducing the amount of carbohydrates you eat. Does this mean you won't get the kind of energy you need for the day? Of course not! It only means that now, your body has to find other possible sources of energy. Do you know where they will be getting that energy? Even before we talk about how to do keto – it's important to first consider why this particular diet works. What actually happens to your body to make you lose weight? As you probably know, the body uses food as an energy source. Everything you eat is turned into energy, so that you can get up and do whatever you need to accomplish for the day. The main energy source is sugar so what happens is that you eat something, the body breaks it down into sugar, and the sugar is processed into energy. Typically, the "sugar" is taken directly from the food you eat so if you eat just the right amount of food, then your body is fueled for the whole day. If you eat too much, then the sugar is stored in your body – hence the accumulation of fat.

But what happens if you eat less food? This is where the Ketogenic Diet comes in. You see, the process of creating sugar from food is usually faster if the food happens to be rich in carbohydrates. Bread, rice, grain, pasta – all of these are carbohydrates and they're the easiest food types to turn into energy.

So here's the situation – you are eating less carbohydrates every day. To keep you energetic, the body breaks down the stored fat and turns them into molecules called ketone bodies. The process of turning the fat into ketone bodies is called "Ketosis" and obviously – this is where the name of the Ketogenic Diet comes from. The ketone bodies take the place of glucose in keeping you energetic. As long as you keep your carbohydrates reduced, the body will keep getting its energy from your body fat.

The Ketogenic Diet is often praised for its simplicity and when you look at it properly, the process is really straightforward. The Science behind the effectivity of the diet is also well-documented, and has been proven multiple times by different medical fields. For example, an article on Diet Review by Harvard provided a lengthy discussion on how the Ketogenic Diet works and why it is so effective for those who choose to use this diet.

But Fat Is the Enemy...Or Is It?

No – fat is NOT the enemy. Unfortunately, years of bad science told us that fat is something you have to avoid – but it's actually a very helpful thing for weight loss! Even before we move forward with this book, we'll have to discuss exactly what "healthy fats" are, and why they're actually the good guys. To do this, we need to make a distinction between the different kinds of fat. You've probably heard of them before and it is a little bit confusing at first. We'll try to go through them as simply as possible:

Saturated fat. This is the kind you want to avoid. They're also called "solid fat" because each molecule is packed with hydrogen atoms. Simply put, it's the kind of fat that can easily cause a blockage in your body. It can raise cholesterol levels and lead to heart problems or a stroke. Saturated fat is something you can find in meat, dairy products, and other processed food items. Now, you're probably wondering: isn't the Ketogenic Diet packed with saturated fat? The answer is: not necessarily. You'll find later in the recipes given that the Ketogenic Diet promotes primarily unsaturated fat or healthy fat. While there are definitely many meat recipes in the list, most of these recipes contain healthy fat sources.

Unsaturated Fat. These are the ones dubbed as healthy fat. They're the kind of fat you find in avocado, nuts, and other ingredients you usually find in Keto-friendly recipes. They're known to lower blood cholesterol and actually come in two types: polyunsaturated and monounsaturated. Both are good for your body but the benefits slightly vary, depending on what you're consuming.

Mexican Lamb Chops

Preparation Time: 10 minutes

Cooking Time: 15 minutes

Servings: 4

Ingredients:

- 4 lamb chops
- 1 tablespoon Mexican seasonings
- 2 tablespoons sesame oil
- 1 teaspoon butter

Directions:

1. Rub the lamb chops with Mexican seasonings.
2. Then melt the butter in the skillet. Add sesame oil.
3. Then add lamb chops and roast them for 7 minutes per side on medium heat.

Nutrition: Calories 323 Fat 14 Fiber 0 Carbs 1.1 Protein 24.1

Tender Lamb Stew

Preparation Time: 10 minutes

Cooking Time: 60 minutes

Servings: 4

Ingredients:

- 1-pound lamb fillet, chopped
- 3 cups of water
- 1 zucchini, chopped
- ½ cup leek, chopped
- 1 teaspoon ground paprika
- 1 teaspoon cayenne pepper
- 1 teaspoon salt
- 1 teaspoon butter

Directions:

1. Put all ingredients in the saucepan. Mix the mixture and close the lid.
2. Cook the stew on medium-low heat for 60 minutes.

Nutrition: Calories 237 Fat 9.5 Fiber 1.1 Carbs 3.8 Protein 32.7

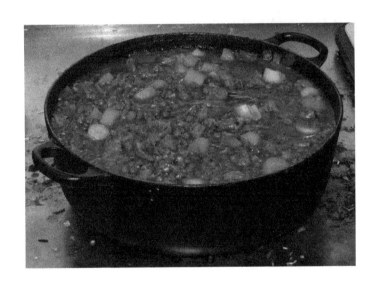

Lime Lamb

Preparation Time: 10 minutes

Cooking Time: 40 minutes

Servings: 4

Ingredients:

- 2 lamb shanks
- ½ lime
- 1 teaspoon salt
- 1 teaspoon Erythritol
- 3 tablespoons butter

Directions:

1. Melt the butter in the saucepan.
2. Add lamb shanks in the hot butter and roast them for 5 minutes per side on the medium heat.
3. Then sprinkle the meat with salt and Erythritol.
4. Close the lid and simmer the meat on low heat for 30 minutes.

Nutrition: Calories 158 Fat 11.8 Fiber 0.2 Carbs 2.1 Protein 12.1

Lamb Saute with Mint and Lemon

Preparation Time: 10 minutes

Cooking Time: 45 minutes

Servings: 4

Ingredients:

- 1-pound lamb fillet
- 1 teaspoon dried mint
- 1 teaspoon lemon zest, grated
- 2 cups of water
- 1 carrot, chopped
- 1 teaspoon keto tomato paste
- 1 teaspoon cayenne pepper

Directions:

1. Chop the lamb fillet roughly and put it in the saucepan.
2. Roast the meat for 2 minutes per side.
3. Add dried mint, lemon zest, carrot, keto tomato paste, and cayenne pepper.
4. Then add water and carefully stir the ingredients.

5. Close the lid and cook the saute on medium heat for 40 minutes.

Nutrition: Calories 220 Fat 8.4 Fiber 0.6 Carbs 2.1 Protein 32.1

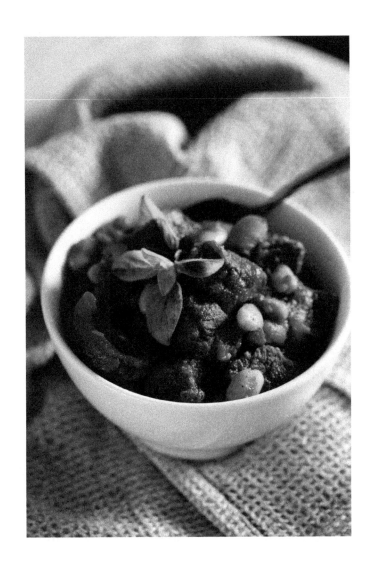

Pancetta Lamb

Preparation Time: 10 minutes

Cooking Time: 35 minutes

Servings: 5

Ingredients:

- 1-pound lamb fillet
- 2 oz. pancetta, sliced
- 1 teaspoon chili powder
- 1 teaspoon ground turmeric
- 1 tablespoon coconut oil

Directions:

1. Cut the lamb fillet into 5 servings.
2. Then mix meat with chili powder and ground turmeric.
3. After this, wrap every lamb fillet with pancetta.
4. Preheat the coconut oil in the skillet.
5. Add meat and roast it for 3 minutes.
6. After this, transfer the meat in the preheated to 360F oven and cook for 30 minutes.

Nutrition: Calories 257 Fat 14.2 Fiber 0.3 Carbs 0.7 Protein 29.8

Sweet Lamb with Oregano

Preparation Time: 10 minutes

Cooking Time: 25 minutes

Servings: 4

Ingredients:

- 1-pound lamb fillet, sliced
- 1 teaspoon dried oregano
- 1 teaspoon Erythritol
- 3 tablespoons butter
- 1 tablespoon apple cider vinegar

Directions:

1. Melt butter in the saucepan.
2. Add dried oregano, Erythritol, and apple cider vinegar. Bring the liquid to boil.
3. Add sliced lamb fillet and roast it for 20 minutes. Stir the meat from time to time.

Nutrition: Calories 289 Fat 17 Fiber 0.2 Carbs 1.5 Protein 32

Veal and Cabbage Salad

Preparation Time: 10 minutes

Cooking Time: 0 minutes

Servings: 4

Ingredients:

- 1-pound veal, boiled, chopped
- 1 cup white cabbage, shredded
- 1 tablespoon olive oil
- 1 teaspoon apple cider vinegar
- 1 teaspoon dried dill
- 1 teaspoon salt

Directions:

1. Put all ingredients in the salad bowl.
2. Carefully mix the salad.

Nutrition: Calories 230 Fat 12.1 Fiber 0.5 Carbs 1.2 Protein 27.9

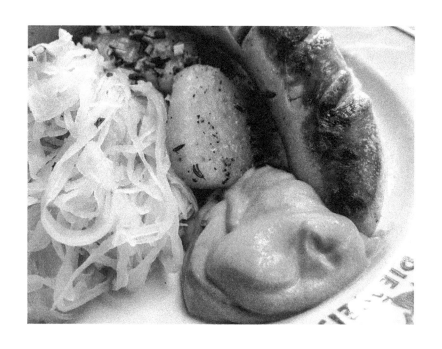

Nutmeg Lamb

Preparation Time: 15 minutes

Cooking Time: 25 minutes

Servings: 4

Ingredients:

- 13 oz. rack of lamb
- 1 teaspoon ground nutmeg
- 1 tablespoon coconut oil
- ½ teaspoon ground black pepper

Directions:

1. Rub the lamb with ground nutmeg and ground black pepper.
2. Then melt the coconut oil in the skillet.
3. Add rack of lamb and roast it on medium heat for 10 minutes per side.

Nutrition: Calories 188 Fat 11.8 Fiber 0.2 Carbs 0.4 Protein 18.8

Oil and Herbs Lamb

Preparation Time: 10 minutes

Cooking Time: 65 minutes

Servings: 4

Ingredients:

- 11 oz. rack of lamb, trimmed
- 3 tablespoons olive oil
- 1 tablespoon Italian seasonings

Directions:

1. Mix the Italian seasonings with olive oil.
2. Then sprinkle the rack of lamb with oily mixture and bake in the oven at 360F for 65 minutes.
3. Slice the cooked lamb.

Nutrition: Calories 232 Fat 18.4 Fiber 0 Carbs 0.4 Protein 15.9

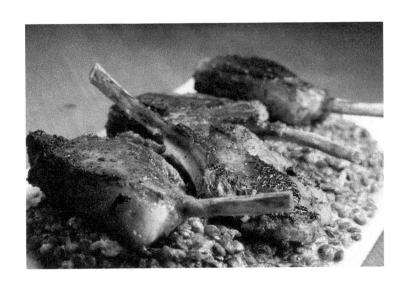

Tomato Lamb Ribs

Preparation Time: 10 minutes

Cooking Time: 30 minutes

Servings: 4

Ingredients:

- 11 oz. lamb ribs, roughly chopped
- 2 teaspoons keto tomato paste
- 2 tablespoons sesame oil
- 1 teaspoon cayenne pepper
- 1 tablespoon apple cider vinegar

Directions:

1. Roast lamb ribs in the sesame oil for 4 minutes per side.
2. Then add keto tomato paste, cayenne pepper, apple cider vinegar, and keto tomato paste.
3. Carefully stir the lamb ribs and close the lid.
4. Cook the lamb ribs on medium heat for 20 minutes.

Nutrition: Calories 222 Fat 14.5 Fiber 0.2 Carbs 0.8 Protein 20.9

SEAFOODS

Salmon with Green Beans

Preparation Time: 10 minutes

Cooking Time: 20 minutes

Servings: 2

Ingredients

- 6 oz. green beans
- 3 oz. unsalted butter
- 2 salmon fillets
- Seasoning:
- ½ tsp garlic powder
- ½ tsp salt
- ½ tsp cracked black pepper

Directions:

1. Take a frying pan, place butter in it and when it starts to melts, add beans and salmon in fillets in it, season with garlic powder, salt, and black pepper, and cook for 8 minutes until salmon is

cooked, turning halfway through and stirring the beans frequently.

2. When done, evenly divide salmon and green beans between two plates and serve.

Nutrition: 352 Calories; 29 g Fats; 19 g Protein; 3.5 g Net Carb; 1.5 g Fiber;

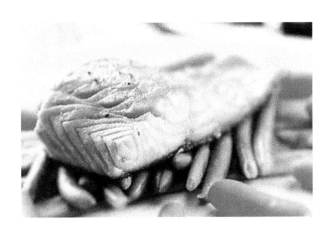

Salmon Sheet pan

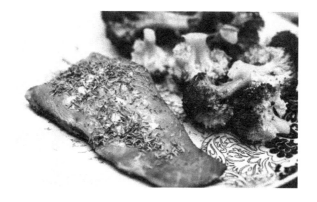

Preparation Time: 10 minutes

Cooking Time: 20 minutes

Servings: 2

Ingredients

- 2 salmon fillets
- 2 oz. cauliflower florets
- 2 oz. broccoli florets
- 1 tsp minced garlic
- 1 tbsp. chopped cilantro
- Seasoning:
- 2 tbsp. coconut oil
- 2/3 tsp salt

- ¼ tsp ground black pepper

Directions:

1. Turn on the oven, then set it to 400 degrees F, and let it preheat.
2. Place oil in a small bowl, add garlic and cilantro, stir well, and microwave for 1 minute or until the oil has melted.
3. Take a rimmed baking sheet, place cauliflower and broccoli florets in it, drizzle with 1 tbsp. of coconut oil mixture, season with 1/3 tsp salt, 1/8 tsp black pepper and bake for 10 minutes.
4. Then push the vegetables to a side, place salmon fillets in the pan, drizzle with remaining coconut oil mixture, season with remaining salt and black pepper on both sides and bake for 10 minutes until salmon is fork-tender.
5. Serve.

Nutrition: 450 Calories; 23.8 g Fats; 36.9 g Protein; 5.9 g Net Carb; 2.4 g Fiber;

Fish with Kale and Olives

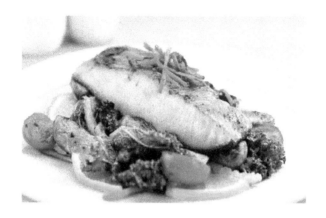

Preparation Time: 5 minutes

Cooking Time: 12 minutes

Servings: 2

Ingredients

- 2 pacific whitening fillets

- 2 oz. chopped kale

- 3 tbsp. coconut oil

- 2 scallion, chopped

- 6 green olives

- Seasoning:

- 1/2 tsp salt

- 1/3 tsp ground black pepper

- 3 drops of liquid stevia

Directions:

1. Take a large skillet pan, place it over medium-high heat, add 4 tbsp. water, then add kale, toss and cook for 2 minutes until leaves are wilted but green.
2. When done, transfer kale to a strainer placed on a bowl and set aside until required.
3. Wipe clean the pan, add 2 tbsp. oil, and wait until it melts.
4. Season fillets with 1/3 tsp salt and ¼ tsp black pepper, place them into the pan skin-side up and cook for 4 minutes per side until fork tender.
5. Transfer fillets to a plate, add remaining oil to the pan, then add scallion and olives and cook for 1 minute.
6. Return kale into the pan, stir until mixed, cook for 1 minute until hot and then season with remaining salt and black pepper.
7. Divide kale mixture between two plates, top with cooked fillets, and then serve.

Nutrition: 454 Calories; 35.8 g Fats; 16 g Protein; 13.5 g Net Carb; 3.5 g Fiber;

Cardamom Salmon

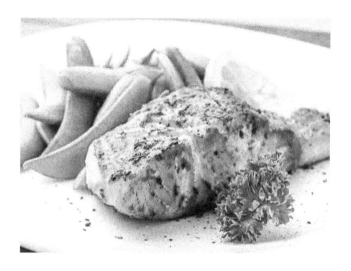

Preparation Time: 5 minutes

Cooking Time: 20 minutes

Servings: 2

Ingredients

- 2 salmon fillets
- ¾ tsp salt
- 2/3 tbsp. ground cardamom
- 1 tbsp. liquid stevia
- 1 ½ tbsp. avocado oil

Directions:

1. Turn on the oven, then set it to 275 degrees F and let it preheat.

2. Meanwhile, prepare the sauce and for this, place oil in a small bowl, and whisk in cardamom and stevia until combined.

3. Take a baking dish, place salmon in it, brush with prepared sauce on all sides, and let it marinate for 20 minutes at room temperature.

4. Then season salmon with salt and bake for 15 to 20 minutes until thoroughly cooked.

5. When done, flake salmon with two forks and then serve.

Nutrition: 143.3 Calories; 10.7 g Fats; 11.8 g Protein; 0 g Net Carb; 0 g Fiber;

Garlic Butter Salmon

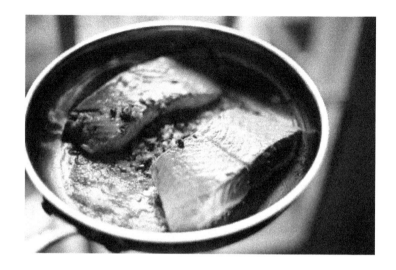

Preparation Time: 10 minutes

Cooking Time: 15 minutes

Servings: 2

Ingredients

- 2 salmon fillets, skinless
- 1 tsp minced garlic
- 1 tbsp. chopped cilantro
- 1 tbsp. unsalted butter
- 2 tbsp. grated cheddar cheese
- Seasoning:

- ½ tsp salt
- ¼ tsp ground black pepper

Directions:

1. Turn on the oven, then set it to 350 degrees F, and let it preheat.

2. Meanwhile, taking a rimmed baking sheet, grease it with oil, place salmon fillets on it, season with salt and black pepper on both sides.

3. Stir together butter, cilantro, and cheese until combined, then coat the mixture on both sides of salmon in an even layer and bake for 15 minutes until thoroughly cooked.

4. Then Turn on the broiler and continue baking the salmon for 2 minutes until the top is golden brown.

5. Serve.

Nutrition: 128 Calories; 4.5 g Fats; 41 g Protein; 1 g Net Carb; 0 g Fiber;

Stir-fry Tuna with Vegetables

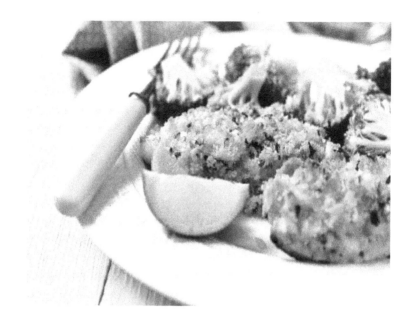

Preparation Time: 5 minutes;

Cooking Time: 15 minutes

Servings: 2

Ingredients

- 4 oz. tuna, packed in water
- 2 oz. broccoli florets
- ½ of red bell pepper, cored, sliced
- ½ tsp minced garlic
- ½ tsp sesame seeds

- Seasoning:
- 1 tbsp. avocado oil
- 2/3 tsp soy sauce
- 2/3 tsp apple cider vinegar
- 3 tbsp. water

Directions:

1. Take a skillet pan, add ½ tbsp. oil and when hot, add bell pepper and cook for 3 minutes until tender-crisp.

2. Then add broccoli floret, drizzle with water and continue cooking for 3 minutes until steamed, covering the pan.

3. Uncover the pan, cook for 2 minutes until all the liquid has evaporated, and then push bell pepper to one side of the pan.

4. Add remaining oil to the other side of the pan, add tuna and cook for 3 minutes until seared on all sides.

5. Then drizzle with soy sauce and vinegar, toss all the ingredients in the pan until mixed and sprinkle with sesame seeds.

6. Serve.

Nutrition: 99.7 Calories; 5.1 g Fats; 11 g Protein; 1.6 g Net Carb; 1 g Fiber;

Baked Fish with Feta and Tomato

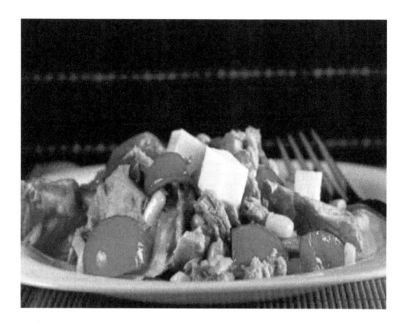

Preparation Time: 5 minutes

Cooking Time: 15 minutes

Servings: 2

Ingredients

- 2 pacific whitening fillets

- 1 scallion, chopped
- 1 Roma tomato, chopped
- 1 tsp fresh oregano
- 1-ounce feta cheese, crumbled
- Seasoning:
- 2 tbsp. avocado oil
- 1/3 tsp salt
- 1/4 tsp ground black pepper
- ¼ crushed red pepper

Directions:

1. Turn on the oven, then set it to 400 degrees F and let it preheat.

2. Take a medium skillet pan, place it over medium heat, add oil and when hot, add scallion and cook for 3 minutes.

3. Add tomatoes, stir in ½ tsp oregano, 1/8 tsp salt, black pepper, red pepper, pour in ¼ cup water and bring it to simmer.

4. Sprinkle remaining salt over fillets, add to the pan, drizzle with remaining oil, and then bake for 10 to 12 minutes until fillets are fork-tender.

5. When done, top fish with remaining oregano and cheese and then serve.

Nutrition: 427.5 Calories; 29.5 g Fats; 26.7 g Protein; 8 g Net Carb; 4 g Fiber;

Chili-glazed Salmon

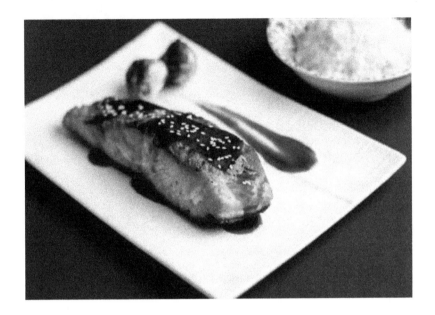

Preparation Time: 5 minutes

Cooking Time: 10 minutes

Servings: 2

Ingredients

- 2 salmon fillets

- 2 tbsp. sweet chili sauce

- 2 tsp chopped chives

- ½ tsp sesame seeds

Directions:

1. Turn on the oven, then set it to 400 degrees F and let it preheat.
2. Meanwhile, place salmon in a shallow dish, add chili sauce and chives and toss until mixed.
3. Transfer prepared salmon onto a baking sheet lined with parchment sheet, drizzle with remaining sauce and bake for 10 minutes until thoroughly cooked.
4. Garnish with sesame seeds and Serve.

Nutrition: 112.5 Calories; 5.6 g Fats; 12 g Protein; 3.4 g Net Carb; 0 g Fiber;

Creamy Tuna, Spinach, and Eggs Plates

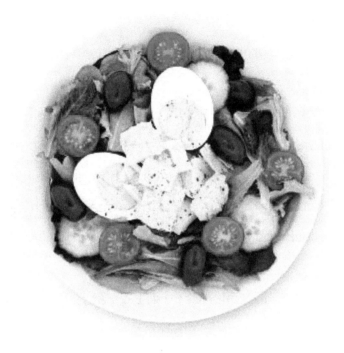

Preparation Time: 5 minutes

Cooking Time: 0 minutes

Servings: 2

Ingredients

- 2 oz. of spinach leaves

- 2 oz. tuna, packed in water
- 2 eggs, boiled
- 4 tbsp. cream cheese, full-fat
- Seasoning:
- ¼ tsp salt
- 1/8 tsp ground black pepper

Directions:

1. Take two plates and evenly distribute spinach and tuna between them.
2. Peel the eggs, cut them into half, and divide them between the plates and then season with salt and black pepper.
3. Serve with cream cheese.

Nutrition: 212 Calories; 14.1 g Fats; 18 g Protein; 1.9 g Net Carb; 1.3 g Fiber;

Tuna and Avocado

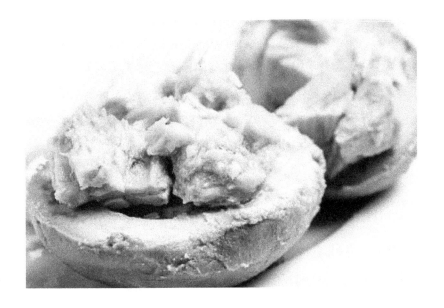

Preparation Time: 5 minutes

Cooking Time: 0 minutes

Servings: 2

Ingredients

- 2 oz. tuna, packed in water
- 1 avocado, pitted
- 8 green olives
- ½ cup mayonnaise, full-fat
- Seasoning:

- 1/3 tsp salt
- 1/4 tsp ground black pepper

Directions:

1. Cut avocado into half, then remove the pit, scoop out the flesh and distribute between two plates.
2. Add tuna and green olives and then season with salt and black pepper.
3. Serve with mayonnaise.

Nutrition: 680 Calories; 65.6 g Fats; 10.2 g Protein; 2.2 g Net Carb; 9.7 g Fiber;

Garlic Oregano Fish

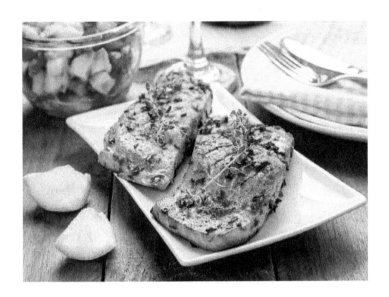

Preparation Time: 5 minutes

Cooking Time: 12 minutes

Servings: 2

Ingredients

- 2 pacific whitening fillets
- 1 tsp minced garlic
- 1 tbsp. butter, unsalted
- 2 tsp dried oregano
- Seasoning:

- 1/3 tsp salt
- 1/4 tsp ground black pepper

Directions:

1. Turn on the oven, then set it to 400 degrees F and let it preheat.
2. Meanwhile, take a small saucepan, place it over low heat, add butter and when it melts, stir in garlic and cook for 1 minute, remove the pan from heat.
3. Season fillets with salt and black pepper, and place them on a baking dish greased with oil.
4. Pour butter mixture over fillets, then sprinkle with oregano and bake for 10 to 12 minutes until thoroughly cooked.
5. Serve.

Nutrition: 199.5 Calories; 7 g Fats; 33.5 g Protein; 0.9 g Net Carb; 0.1 g Fiber;

Bacon wrapped Salmon

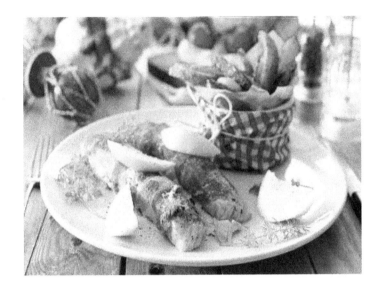

Preparation Time: 5 minutes

Cooking Time: 10 minutes

Servings: 2

Ingredients

- 2 salmon fillets, cut into four pieces
- 4 slices of bacon
- 2 tsp avocado oil
- 2 tbsp. mayonnaise
- Seasoning:

- ½ tsp salt
- ½ tsp ground black pepper

Directions:

1. Turn on the oven, then set it to 375 degrees F and let it preheat.

2. Meanwhile, place a skillet pan, place it over medium-high heat, add oil and let it heat.

3. Season salmon fillets with salt and black pepper, wrap each salmon fillet with a bacon slice, then add to the pan and cook for 4 minutes, turning halfway through.

4. Then transfer skillet pan containing salmon into the oven and cook salmon for 5 minutes until thoroughly cooked.

5. Serve salmon with mayonnaise

Nutrition: 190.7 Calories; 16.5 g Fats; 10.5 g Protein; 0 g Net Carb; 0 g Fiber;

Fish and Spinach Plate

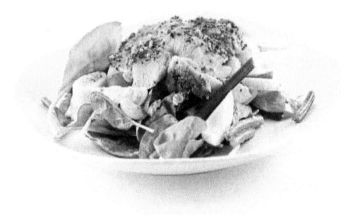

Preparation Time: 10 minutes

Cooking Time: 10 minutes

Servings: 2

Ingredients

- 2 pacific whitening fillets
- 2 oz. spinach
- ½ cup mayonnaise
- 1 tbsp. avocado oil
- 1 tbsp. unsalted butter

- Seasoning:
- 1/2 tsp salt
- 1/3 tsp ground black pepper

Directions:

1. Take a frying pan, place it over medium heat, add butter and wait until it melts.
2. Season fillets with 1/3 tsp salt and ¼ tsp black pepper, add to the pan, and cook for 5 minutes per side until golden brown and thoroughly cooked.
3. Transfer fillets to two plates, then distribute spinach among them, drizzle with oil and season with remaining salt and black pepper.
4. Serve with mayonnaise.

Nutrition: 389 Calories; 34 g Fats; 7.7 g Protein; 10.6 g Net Carb; 2 g Fiber

Fish and Egg Plate

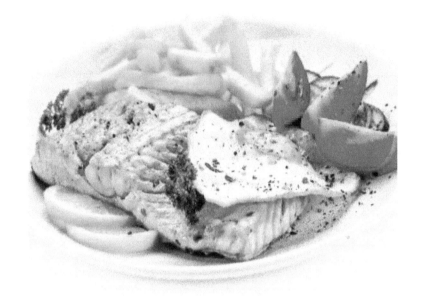

Preparation Time: 5 minutes;

Cooking Time: 10 minutes

Servings: 2

Ingredients

- 2 eggs
- 1 tbsp. butter, unsalted
- 2 pacific whitening fillets
- ½ oz. chopped lettuce
- 1 scallion, chopped

- Seasoning:
- 3 tbsp. avocado oil
- 1/3 tsp salt
- 1/3 tsp ground black pepper

Directions:

1. Cook the eggs and for this, take a frying pan, place it over medium heat, add butter and when it melts, crack the egg in the pan and cook for 2 to 3 minutes until fried to desired liking.

2. Transfer fried egg to a plate and then cook the remaining egg in the same manner.

3. Meanwhile, season fish fillets with ¼ tsp each of salt and black pepper.

4. When eggs have fried, sprinkle salt and black pepper on them, then add 1 tbsp. oil into the frying pan, add fillets and cook for 4 minutes per side until thoroughly cooked.

5. When done, distribute fillets to the plate, add lettuce and scallion, drizzle with remaining oil, and then serve.

Herb Crusted Tilapia

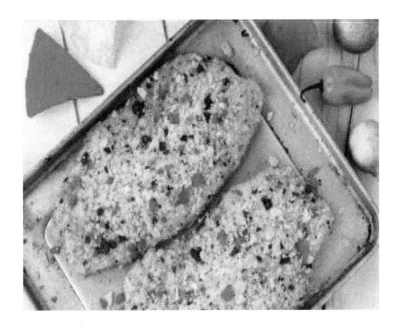

Preparation Time: 5 minutes

Cooking Time: 10 minutes

Servings: 2

Ingredients

- 2 fillets of tilapia
- ½ tsp garlic powder
- ½ tsp Italian seasoning
- ½ tsp dried parsley

- 1/3 tsp salt
- Seasoning:
- 2 tbsp. melted butter, unsalted
- 1 tbsp. avocado oil

Directions:

1. Turn on the broiler and then let it preheat.
2. Meanwhile, take a small bowl, place melted butter in it, stir in oil and garlic powder until mixed, and then brush this mixture over tilapia fillets.
3. Stir together remaining spices and then sprinkle them generously on tilapia until well coated.
4. Place seasoned tilapia in a baking pan, place the pan under the broiler and then bake for 10 minutes until tender and golden, brushing with garlic-butter every 2 minutes.
5. Serve.

Nutrition: 520 Calories; 35 g Fats; 36.2 g Protein; 13.6 g Net Carb; 0.6 g Fiber;

Smoked Salmon Fat Bombs

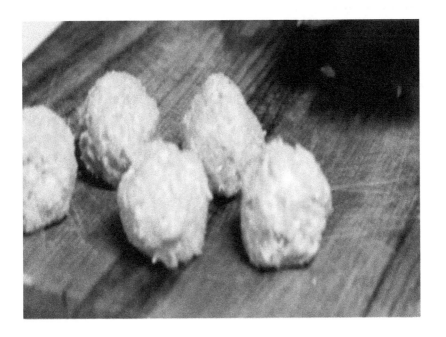

Preparation Time: 5 minutes

Cooking Time: 0 minutes

Servings: 2

Ingredients

- 2 tbsp. cream cheese, softened
- 1 ounce smoked salmon
- 2 tsp bagel seasoning

Directions:

1. Take a medium bowl, place cream cheese and salmon in it, and stir until well combined.

2. Shape the mixture into bowls, roll them into bagel seasoning and then serve.

Nutrition: 65 Calories; 4.8 g Fats; 4 g Protein; 0.5 g Net Carb; 0 g Fiber;

Shrimp Deviled Eggs

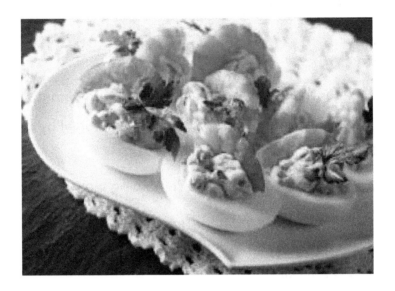

Preparation Time: 5 minutes

Cooking Time: 0 minutes

Servings: 2

Ingredients

- 2 eggs, boiled
- 2 oz. shrimps, cooked, chopped
- ½ tsp tabasco sauce
- ½ tsp mustard paste
- 2 tbsp. mayonnaise

- Seasoning:
- 1/8 tsp salt
- 1/8 tsp ground black pepper

Directions:

1. Peel the boiled eggs, then slice in half lengthwise and transfer egg yolks to a medium bowl by using a spoon.
2. Mash the egg yolk, add remaining ingredients and stir until well combined.
3. Spoon the egg yolk mixture into egg whites, and then serve.

Nutrition: 210 Calories; 16.4 g Fats; 14 g Protein; 1 g Net Carb; 0.1 g Fiber;

Tuna Melt Jalapeno Peppers

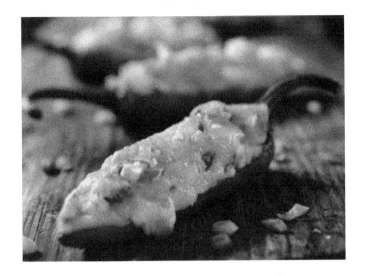

Preparation Time: 5 minutes

Cooking Time: 10 minutes

Servings: 2

Ingredients

- 4 jalapeno peppers
- 1-ounce tuna, packed in water
- 1-ounce cream cheese softened
- 1 tbsp. grated parmesan cheese
- 1 tbsp. grated mozzarella cheese
- Seasoning:

- 1 tsp chopped dill pickles
- 1 green onion, green part sliced only

Directions:

1. Turn on the oven, then set it to 400 degrees F and let it preheat.
2. Prepare the peppers and for this, cut each pepper in half lengthwise and remove seeds and stem.
3. Take a small bowl, place tuna in it, add remaining ingredients except for cheeses, and then stir until combined.
4. Spoon tuna mixture into peppers, sprinkle cheeses on top, and then bake for 7 to 10 minutes until cheese has turned golden brown.
5. Serve.

Nutrition: 104 Calories; 6.2 g Fats; 7 g Protein; 2.1 g Net Carb; 1.1 g Fiber;

Salmon Cucumber Rolls

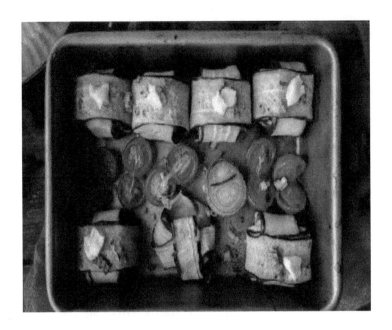

Preparation Time: 15 minutes

Cooking Time: 0 minutes

Servings: 2

Ingredients

- 1 large cucumber
- 2 oz. smoked salmon
- 4 tbsp. mayonnaise
- 1 tsp sesame seeds

- Seasoning:
- ¼ tsp salt
- ¼ tsp ground black pepper

Directions:

1. Trim the ends of the cucumber, cut it into slices by using a vegetable peeler, and then place half of the cucumber slices in a dish.

2. Cover with paper towels, layer with remaining cucumber slices, top with paper towels, and let them refrigerate for 5 minutes.

3. Meanwhile, take a medium bowl, place salmon in it, add mayonnaise, season with salt and black pepper, and then stir until well combined.

4. Remove cucumber slices from the refrigerator, place salmon on one side of each cucumber slice, and then roll tightly.

5. Repeat with remaining cucumber, sprinkle with sesame seeds and then serve.

Nutrition: 269 Calories; 24 g Fats; 6.7 g Protein; 4 g Net Carb; 2 g Fiber;

Sesame Tuna Salad

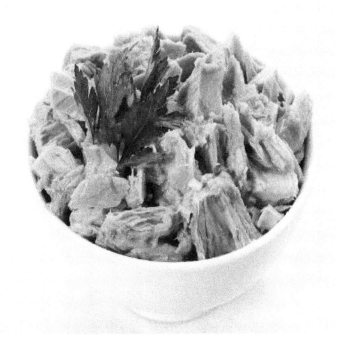

Preparation Time: 35 minutes

Cooking Time: 0 minutes

Servings: 2

Ingredients

- 6 oz. of tuna in water

- ½ tbsp. chili-garlic paste

- ½ tbsp. black sesame seeds, toasted

- 2 tbsp. mayonnaise
- 1 tbsp. sesame oil
- Seasoning:
- 1/8 tsp red pepper flakes

Directions:

1. Take a medium bowl, all the ingredients for the salad in it except for tuna, and then stir until well combined.
2. Fold in tuna until mixed and then refrigerator for 30 minutes.
3. Serve.

Nutrition: 322 Calories; 25.4 g Fats; 17.7 g Protein; 2.6 g Net Carb; 3 g Fiber;

SOUP AND STEW

Chicken Enchilada Soup

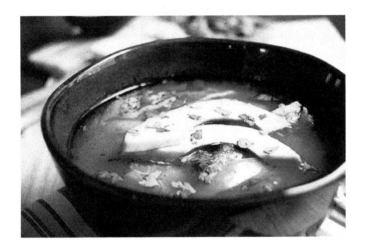

Preparation Time: 10 minutes

Cooking Time: 45 minutes

Servings: 4

Ingredients:

- ½ c. fresh cilantro, chopped

- 1 ¼ tsp. chili powder

- 1 c. fresh tomatoes, diced

- 1 med. yellow onion, diced
- 1 sm. red bell pepper, diced
- 1 tbsp. cumin, ground
- 1 tbsp. extra virgin olive oil
- 1 tbsp. lime juice, fresh
- 1 tsp. dried oregano
- 2 cloves garlic, minced
- 2 lg. stalks celery, diced
- 4 c. chicken broth
- 8 oz. chicken thighs, boneless & skinless, shredded
- 8 oz. cream cheese, softened

Direction:

1. In a pot over medium heat, warm olive oil.
2. Once hot, add celery, red pepper, onion, and garlic. Cook for about 3 minutes or until shiny.
3. Stir the tomatoes into the pot and let cook for another 2 minutes.
4. Add seasonings to the pot, stir in chicken broth and bring to a boil.
5. Once boiling, drop the heat down to low and allow to simmer for 20 minutes.

6. Once simmered, add the cream cheese and allow the soup to return to a boil. *

7. Drop the heat once again and allow to simmer for another 20 minutes.

8. Stir the shredded chicken into the soup along with the lime juice and the cilantro.

9. Spoon into bowls and serve hot!

Nutrition: Calories: 420 Carbohydrates: 9 grams Fat: 29.5 grams Protein: 27 grams

Buffalo Chicken Soup

Preparation Time: 20 minutes

Cooking Time: 20 minutes

Servings: 4

Ingredients:

- 4 med. stalks celery, diced
- 2 med. carrots, diced
- 4 chicken breasts, boneless & skinless
- 6 tbsp. butter
- 1 qt. chicken broth
- 2 oz. cream cheese
- ½ c. heavy cream
- ½ c. buffalo sauce 1 tsp. sea salt
- ½ tsp. thyme, dried
- For garnish:
- Sour cream
- Green onions, thinly sliced
- Bleu cheese crumbles

Direction:

1. Set a large pot to warm over medium heat with the olive oil in it.

2. Cook celery and carrot until shiny and tender. Add chicken breasts to the pot and cover. Allow to cook about five to six minutes per side. Once the chicken has cooked and formed some caramelization on each side, remove it from the pot.

3. Shred the chicken breasts and set aside. Pour the chicken broth into the pot with the carrots and celery, then stir in the cream, butter, and cream cheese. * Bring the pot to a boil, then add chicken back to the pot. Stir buffalo sauce into the mix and combine completely. Feel free to increase or decrease as desired.

4. Add seasonings, stir, and drop the heat to low. Allow the soup to simmer for 15 to 20 minutes, or until all the flavors have fully combined. Serve hot with a garnish of sour cream, bleu cheese crumbles, and sliced green onion!

Nutrition: Calories: 563 Carbohydrates: 4 grams Fat: 32.5 grams Protein: 57 grams

The Salsa

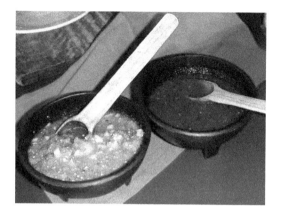

Preparation Time: 20 minutes

Cooking Time: 40 minutes

Servings: 1

Ingredients

- One small tomato
- One Thai chili, thinly sliced.
- One teaspoon of caper, fine cut
- Parsley - 2 teaspoons fine cut
- 1/4 of a lemon's juice

Directions

1. Remove the eye from the tomato to make the salsa and slice it finely, ensuring that the fluid

remains in as much as possible. Combine chile, capers, lemon juice and parsley. You might mix it all in, but the end product is a little different.

2. Oven to 220 degrees Celsius (425 ° F), in one teaspoon, marinate the chicken breast with a little oil and lemon juice. Leave for five to ten minutes.

3. Then add the marinated chicken and cook on either side for about a minute, until pale golden, transfer to the oven (on a baking tray, if your pan is not ovenproof), 8 to 10 minutes or until cooked. Remove from the oven, cover with tape, and wait until eaten for five minutes.

4. Cook the kale for 5 minutes in a steamer in the meantime, add a little butter, fry the red onions and the ginger and then mix in the fluffy but not browned mix.

5. Cook the buckwheat with the remaining teaspoon of turmeric according to the package instructions. Eat rice, tomatoes and salsa. Eat together.

Nutrition: Calories: 104, Sodium: 33 mg, Dietary Fibre: 1.6 g, Total Fat: 4.3 g, Total Carbs: 15.3 g,Protein: 1.3 g.

Ras-el-Hanout hot sauce

Preparation Time: 10 minutes

Cooking Time: 10 minutes

Servings: 2

Ingredients:

- Olive oil

- Lemon slices (juice)

- Teaspoon honey

- 1½ teaspoons Ras el Hanout

- 1/ 2 red peppers, prepare:

Directions:

1. Remove the seeds from the pepper.

2. Chopped peppers.

3. Put pepper in a bowl filled with lemon juice, honey and Ras-ElHanout and mix.

4. Then add olive oil drop by drop while continuing to mix. Sweet and Sour Pot:

Nutrition: Calories: 1495, Sodium: 33 mg, Dietary Fibre: 1.6 g, Total Fat: 3.1 g, Total Carbs: 16.5 g,Protein: 1.3 g.

Teriyaki Sauce

Preparation Time: 10 minutes

Cooking Time: 30 minutes

Servings: 1

Ingredients

- 7fl oz. soy sauce
- 7fl oz. pineapple juice
- 1 teaspoon red wine vinegar
- 1-inch chunk of fresh ginger root, peeled and chopped
- 2 cloves of garlic

Directions

1. Place the ingredients into a saucepan, bring them to the boil, reduce the heat and simmer for 10 minutes. Let it cool then remove the garlic and ginger. Store it in a container in the fridge until ready to use. Use as a marinade for meat, fish and tofu dishes.

Nutrition: Calories: 267, Sodium: 33 mg, Dietary Fibre: 1.2 g, Total Fat: 4.3 g, Total Carbs: 16.2 g, Protein: 1.3 g.

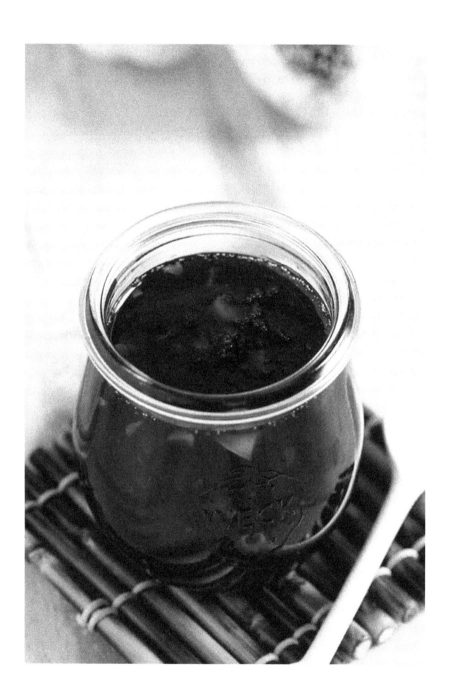

Garlic Vinaigrette

Preparation Time: 10 minutes

Cooking Time: 30 minutes

Servings: 1

Ingredients

- 1 clove garlic, crushed
- 4 tablespoons olive oil
- 1 tablespoon lemon juice
- Freshly ground black pepper

Directions

1. Simply mix all of the ingredients together. It can either be stored or used straight away.

Nutrition: Calories: 104, Sodium: 35 mg, Dietary Fibre: 1.3 g, Total Fat: 3.1 g, Total Carbs: 16.2 g,Protein: 1.3 g.

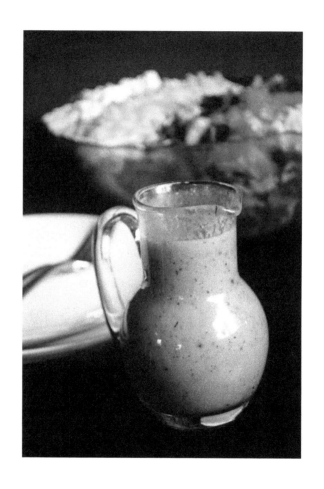

Lemon Caper Pesto

Preparation Time: 10 minutes

Cooking Time: 10 minutes

Servings: 1

Ingredients

- 6 tablespoons fresh parsley leaves
- 3 cloves of garlic
- 2 tablespoons capers
- 2oz cashew nuts
- 2 tablespoons olive oil
- 1 tablespoon lemon juice

Directions

1. Place all of the ingredients into a food processor and blitz until smooth. Add a little extra oil if necessary. Serve with pasta, vegetables or meat dishes.

Nutrition: Calories: 250, Sodium: 32 mg, Dietary Fibre: 1.6 g, Total Fat: 4.1 g, Total Carbs: 16.4 g, Protein: 1.5 g.

Parsley Pesto

Preparation Time: 10 minutes

Cooking Time: 10 minutes

Servings: 1

Ingredients

- 3oz Parmesan cheese, finely grated
- 2oz pine nuts
- 6 tablespoons fresh parsley leaves, chopped
- 2 cloves of garlic
- 2 tablespoons olive oil

Direction

1. Put all of the ingredients into a food processor or blend until you have a smooth paste.

Nutrition: Calories: 104, Sodium: 32 mg, Dietary Fibre: 1.6 g, Total Fat: 4.3 g, Total Carbs: 16.2 g,Protein: 1.3 g.

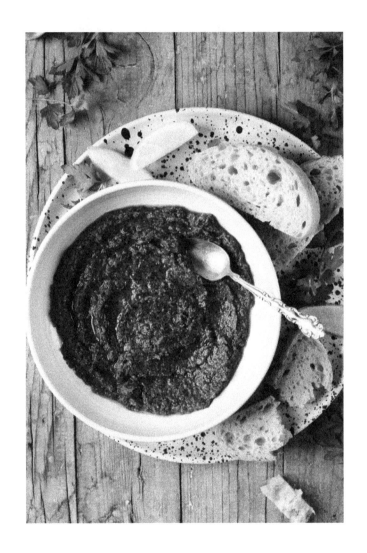

Slow Cooker Taco Soup

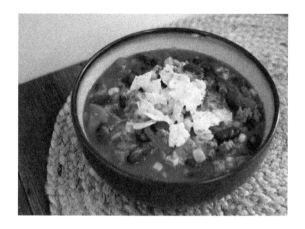

Preparation Time: 10 minutes

Cooking Time: 2 hours

Servings: 8

Ingredients:

- ¼ c. sour cream
- ½ c. cheddar cheese, shredded
- 2 c. diced tomatoes
- 2 lbs. ground beef
- 3 tbsp. taco seasoning*
- 4 c. chicken broth
- 8 oz. cream cheese, cubed**

Direction:

1. Heat a medium saucepan over medium heat and brown the beef.
2. Drain the fat from the beef and then place it into the slow cooker.
3. Add the cream cheese cubes, taco seasoning, and diced tomatoes into the slow cooker.
4. Add the chicken broth, cover and leave to cook on high for two hours.
5. Once the timer is up, stir all the ingredients and spoon the soup into bowls.
6. Serve hot with sour cream and shredded cheese on top!
7. *Check the label! Make sure that the taco seasoning you buy doesn't contain hidden sugars or starches.
8. **Cream cheese is easier to cut when it's very cold and if you carefully spread a little bit of olive oil on the blade of the knife!

Nutrition: Calories: 505 Carbohydrates: 8.5 grams Fat: 31.5 grams Protein: 43.5 grams

Walnut Vinaigrette

Preparation Time: 10 minutes

Cooking Time: 10 minutes

Servings: 1

Ingredients

- 1 clove garlic, finely chopped
- 6 tablespoons olive oil
- 3 tablespoons red wine vinegar
- 1 tablespoon walnut oil
- Sea salt
- Freshly ground black pepper

Directions

1. Combine all of the ingredients in a bowl or container and season with salt and pepper. Use immediately or store in the fridge.

Nutrition: Calories: 109, Sodium: 33 mg, Dietary Fibre: 1.6 g, Total Fat: 4.3 g, Total Carbs: 16.4 g,Protein: 1.6 g.

Turmeric & Lemon Dressing

Preparation Time: 10 minutes

Cooking Time: 30 minutes

Servings: 1

Ingredients

- 1 teaspoon turmeric
- 4 tablespoons olive oil
- Juice of 1 lemon

Directions

1. Combine all the ingredients in bowl and serve with salads. Eat straight away.

Nutrition: Calories: 125, Sodium: 32 mg, Dietary Fibre: 1.6 g, Total Fat: 3.3 g, Total Carbs: 16.3 g,Protein: 1.5 g.

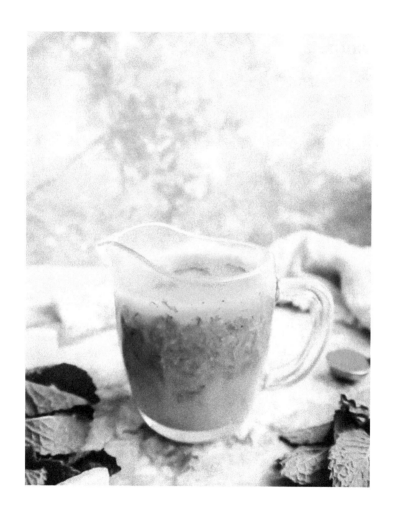

Walnut & Mint Pesto

Preparation Time: 10 minutes

Cooking Time: 10 minutes

Servings: 1

Ingredients

- 6 tablespoons fresh mint leaves
- 2oz walnuts
- 2 cloves of garlic
- 3½oz Parmesan cheese
- 1 tablespoon lemon juice

Direction

1. Put all the ingredients into a food processor and blend until it becomes a smooth paste.

Nutrition: Calories: 99, Sodium: 33 mg, Dietary Fibre: 1.6 g, Total Fat: 4.4 g, Total Carbs: 16.4 g,Protein: 1.6 g.

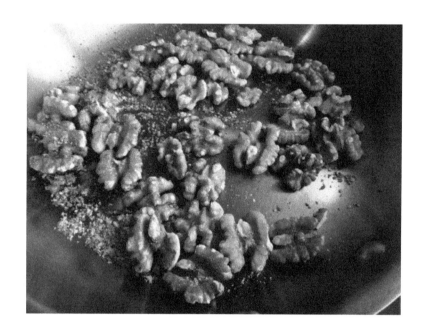

Wedding Soup

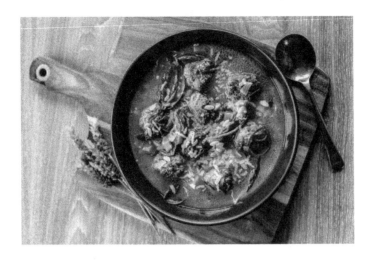

Preparation Time: 5 minutes

Cooking Time: 10 minutes

Servings: 4

Ingredients:

- ½ c. almond flour
- ½ c. parmesan cheese, grated
- ½ sm. yellow onion, diced
- 1 lb. ground beef
- 1 lg. egg, beaten
- 1 tsp. Italian seasoning
- 1 tsp. oregano, fresh & chopped

- 1 tsp. thyme, fresh & chopped
- 2 c. baby leaf spinach, fresh
- 2 c. cauliflower, riced
- 2 med. stalks celery, diced
- 2 tbsp. extra virgin olive oil
- 3 cloves garlic, minced
- 6 c. chicken broth
- Sea salt & pepper to taste

Direction:

1. In a large mixing bowl, combine almond flour, parmesan cheese, ground beef, egg, salt, pepper, and Italian seasoning. Mix thoroughly by band

2. Shape the meat mixture into one-inch meatballs, cover, and refrigerate until ready to cook.

3. In a large saucepan over medium heat, warm the olive oil.

4. Once the oil is hot, stir the celery and onion into the pan and season to taste with salt and pepper.

5. Stirring often, bring the onion and celery to a lightly cooked state, about six or seven minutes.

6. Add the garlic to the pan, stir to combine, and allow to cook for one more minute.

7. Stir chicken broth, fresh oregano, and the fresh thyme into the pan and stir to combine.

8. Bring the mixture to a boil.

9. Drop the heat to low and allow to simmer for about ten minutes before adding cauliflower and meatballs to it.

10.Allow to cook for about five minutes or until the meatballs are cooked all the way through.

11.Add the spinach to the soup and stir in for about one to two minutes, or until it's sufficiently wilted.

12.Add seasoning as is needed.

13.Serve hot!

Nutrition: Calories: 420 Carbohydrates: 4 grams Fat: 26 grams Protein: 6.5 grams

SOUP RECIPES

Vinaigrette

Preparation Time: 10 minutes

Cooking Time: 10 minutes

Servings: 2

Ingredients:

- A teaspoon of yellow mustard
- A spoon of white wine vinegar
- 1 Teaspoon of honey
- 165 ml of prepared olive oil:

Directions

1. Mix mustard, vinegar and honey in a bowl.
2. Add a small amount of olive oil and stir until the vinegar thickens.
3. Season with salt and pepper.

Nutrition: Calories: 1495, Sodium: 33 mg, Dietary Fibre: 1.4 g, Total Fat: 4.3 g, Total Carbs: 16.2 g, Protein: 1.5 g.

Mexican Pork Stew

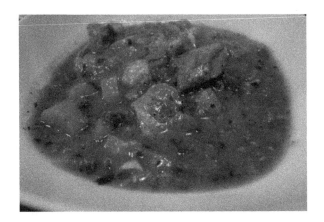

Preparation Time: 15 minutes

Cooking Time: 2 hours 10 minutes

Servings: 1

Ingredients:

- 3 tbsp. unsalted butter
- 2½ lb. boneless pork ribs, cut into ¾-inch cubes
- 1 large yellow onion, chopped
- 4 garlic cloves, crushed
- 1½ C. homemade chicken broth
- 2 (10-oz.) cans sugar-free diced tomatoes
- 1 C. canned roasted poblano chiles
- 2 tsp. dried oregano

- 1 tsp. ground cumin
- Salt, to taste
- ¼ C. fresh cilantro, chopped
- 2 tbsp. fresh lime juice

Direction:

1. In a large pan, melt the butter over medium-high heat and cook the pork, onions and garlic for about 5 minutes or until browned.
2. Add the broth and scrape up the browned bits.
3. Add the tomatoes, poblano chiles, oregano, cumin, and salt and bring to a boil.
4. Reduce the heat to medium-low and simmer, covered for about 2 hours.
5. Stir in the fresh cilantro and lime juice and remove from heat.
6. Serve hot.

Nutrition: Calories: 288 Carbohydrates: 8.8g Protein: 39.6g Fat: 10.1g Sugar: 4g Sodium: 283mgFiber: 2.8g

Curry Soup

Preparation Time: 25 minutes

Cooking Time: 20 minutes

Servings: 4

Ingredients:

- ¾ tsp. cumin
- ¼ c. pumpkin seeds, raw
- ½ tsp. garlic powder
- ½ tsp. paprika ½ tsp. sea salt
- 1 c. coconut milk, unsweetened
- 1 clove garlic, minced
- 1 med. onion, diced
- 2 c. carrots, chopped
- 2 tbsp. curry powder
- 3 c. cauliflower, riced
- 3 tbsp. extra virgin olive oil, divided
- 4 c. kale, chopped
- 4 c. vegetable broth
- Sea salt & pepper to taste

Direction:

1. Hear a large saute pan over medium heat with 2 tablespoons of olive oil. Once the oil is hot, add the rice cauliflower to the pan along with the curry powder, cumin, salt, paprika, and garlic powder. Stir thoroughly to combine.
2. While cooking, stir occasionally. Once the cauliflower is warmed through, remove it from the heat.
3. In a large pot over medium heat, add the remainder of your olive oil. Once it's hot, add the onion and allow it to cook for about four minutes. Add the garlic, then cook for about another two minutes.
4. To the large pot, add the broth, kale, carrots, and cauliflower. Stir to thoroughly incorporate.
5. Allow the mixture to come to a boil, drop the heat to low, and allow the soup to simmer for about 15 minutes.
6. Stir the coconut milk into the mixture along with salt and pepper to taste.
7. Garnish with pumpkin seeds and serve hot!

Nutrition: Calories: 274 Carbs: 11 grams Fat: 19 grams Protein: 15 grams

Winter Comfort stew

Preparation Time: 15 minutes

Cooking Time: 50 minutes

Servings: 6

Ingredients:

- 2 tbsp. olive oil
- 1 small yellow onion, chopped
- 2 garlic cloves, chopped
- 2 lb. grass-fed beef chuck, cut into 1-inch cubes
- 1 (14-oz.) can sugar-free crushed tomatoes
- 2 tsp. ground allspice
- 1½ tsp. red pepper flakes
- ½ C. homemade beef broth
- 6 oz. green olives, pitted
- 8 oz. fresh baby spinach
- 2 tbsp. fresh lemon juice
- Salt and freshly ground black pepper, to taste
- ¼ C. fresh cilantro, chopped

Direction:

1. In a pan, heat the oil in a pan over high heat and sauté the onion and garlic for about 2-3 minutes.

2. Add the beef and cook for about 3-4 minutes or until browned, stirring frequently.
3. Add the tomatoes, spices and broth and bring to a boil.
4. Reduce the heat to low and simmer, covered for about 30-40 minutes or until desired doneness of the beef.
5. Stir in the olives and spinach and simmer for about 2-3 minutes.
6. Stir in the lemon juice, salt and black pepper and remove from the heat.
7. Serve hot with the garnishing of cilantro.

Nutrition: Calories: 388 Carbohydrates: 8g Protein: 485g Fat: 17.7g Sugar: 2.6g Sodium: 473mgFiber: 3.1g

Hungarian Pork Stew

Preparation Time: 15 minutes

Cooking Time: 2 hours 20 minutes

Servings: 10

Ingredients:

- 3 tbsp. olive oil
- 3½ lb. pork shoulder, cut into 4 portions
- 1 tbsp. butter
- 2 medium onions, chopped
- 16 oz. tomatoes, crushed
- 5 garlic cloves, crushed
- 2 Hungarian wax peppers, chopped
- 3 tbsp. Hungarian Sweet paprika
- 1 tbsp. smoked paprika
- 1 tsp. hot paprika
- ½ tsp. caraway seeds
- 1 bay leaf
- 1 C. homemade chicken broth
- 1 packet unflavored gelatin
- 2 tbsp. fresh lemon juice
- Pinch of xanthan gum
- Salt and freshly ground black pepper, to taste

Directions:

1. In a heavy-bottomed pan, heat 1 tbsp. of oil over high heat and sear the pork for about 2-3 minutes or until browned.
2. Transfer the pork onto a plate and cut into bite-sized pieces.
3. In the same pan, heat 1 tbsp. of oil and butter over medium-low heat and sauté the onions for about 5-6 minutes.
4. With a slotted spoon transfer the onion into a bowl.
5. In the same pan, add the tomatoes and cook for about 3-4 minutes, without stirring.
6. Meanwhile, in a small frying pan, heat the remaining oil over-low heat and sauté the garlic, wax peppers, all kinds of paprika and caraway seeds for about 20-30 seconds.
7. Remove from the heat and set aside.
8. In a small bowl, mix together the gelatin and broth.

9. In the large pan, add the cooked pork, garlic mixture, gelatin mixture and bay leaf and bring t0 a gentle boil.

10. Reduce the heat to low and simmer, covered for about 2 hours.

11. Stir in the xanthan gum and simmer for about 3-5 minutes.

12. Stir in the lemon juice, salt and black pepper and remove from the heat.

13. Serve hot.

Nutrition: Calories: 529 Carbohydrates: 5.8g Protein: 38.9g Fat: 38.5g Sugar: 2.6g Sodium: 216mgFiber: 2.1g

Weekend Dinner Stew

Preparation Time: 15 minutes

Cooking Time: 55 minutes

Servings: 6

Ingredients:

- 1½ lb. grass-fed beef stew meat, trimmed and cubed into 1-inch size
- Salt and freshly ground black pepper, to taste
- 1 tbsp. olive oil
- 1 C. homemade tomato puree
- 4 C. homemade beef broth
- 2 C. zucchini, chopped
- 2 celery ribs, sliced
- ½ C. carrots, peeled and sliced
- 2 garlic cloves, minced
- ½ tbsp. dried thyme
- 1 tsp. dried parsley
- 1 tsp. dried rosemary
- 1 tbsp. paprika
- 1 tsp. onion powder
- 1 tsp. garlic powder

Direction:

1. In a large bowl, add the beef cubes, salt and black pepper and toss to coat well.

2. In a large pan, heat the oil over medium-high heat and cook the beef cubes for about 4-5 minutes or until browned.

3. Add the remaining ingredients and stir to combine.

4. Increase the heat to high and bring to a boil.

5. Reduce the heat to low and simmer, covered for about 40-50 minutes.

6. Stir in the salt and black pepper and remove from the heat.

7. Serve hot.

Nutrition: Calories: 293 Carbohydrates: 8g Protein: 9.3g Fat: 10.7g Sugar: 4g Sodium: 223mg Fiber: 2.3g

Yellow Chicken Soup

Preparation Time: 15 minutes

Cooking Time: 25 minutes

Servings: 5

Ingredients:

- 2½ tsp. ground turmeric
- 1½ tsp. ground cumin
- 1/8 tsp cayenne pepper
- 2 tbsp. butter, divided
- 1 small yellow onion, chopped
- 2 C. cauliflower, chopped
- 2 C. broccoli, chopped
- 4 C. homemade chicken broth
- 1½ C. water
- 1 tsp. fresh ginger root, grated
- 1 bay leaf
- 2 C. Swiss chard, stemmed and chopped finely
- ½ C. unsweetened coconut milk
- 3 (4-oz.) grass-fed boneless, skinless chicken thighs, cut into bite-size pieces
- 2 tbsp. fresh lime juice

Direction:

1. In a small bowl, mix together the turmeric, cumin and cayenne pepper and set aside.

2. Ina large pan, melt 1 tbsp. of the butter over medium heat and sauté the onion for about 3-4 minutes.

3. Add the cauliflower, broccoli and half of the spice mixture and cook for another 3-4 minutes.

4. Add the broth, water, ginger and bay leaf and bring to a boil.

5. Reduce the heat to low and simmer for about 8-10 minutes.

6. Stir in the Swiss chard and coconut milk and cook for about 1-2 minutes.

7. Meanwhile, in a large skillet, melt the remaining butter over medium heat and sear the chicken pieces for about 5 minutes.

8. Stir in the remaining spice mix and cook for about 5 minutes, stirring frequently.

9. Transfer the soup into serving bowls and top with the chicken pieces.

10. Drizzle with lime juice and serve.

Nutrition: Calories: 258 Carbohydrates: 8.4g Protein: 18.4g Fat: 16.8g Sugar: 3g Sodium: 753mgFiber: 2.9g

Ideal Cold Weather Stew

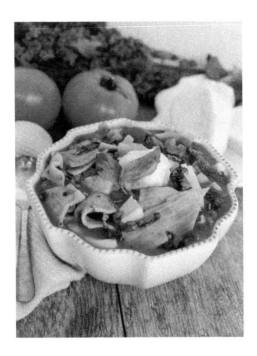

Preparation Time: 20 minutes

Cooking Time: 2 hours 40 minutes

Servings: 6

Ingredients:

- 3 tbsp. olive oil, divided
- 8 oz. fresh mushrooms, quartered
- 1¼ lb. grass-fed beef chuck roast, trimmed and cubed into 1-inch size

- 2 tbsp. tomato paste
- ½ tsp. dried thyme
- 1 bay leaf
- 5 C. homemade beef broth
- 6 oz. celery root, peeled and cubed
- 4 oz. yellow onions, chopped roughly
- 3 oz. carrot, peeled and sliced
- 2 garlic cloves, sliced
- Salt and freshly ground black pepper, to taste

Direction:

1. In a Dutch oven, heat 1 tbsp. of the oil over medium heat and cook the mushrooms for about 2 minutes, without stirring.
2. Stir the mushroom and cook for about 2 minutes more.
3. With a slotted spoon, transfer the mushroom onto a plate.
4. In the same pan, heat the remaining oil over medium-high heat and sear the beef cubes for about 4-5 minutes.
5. Stir in the tomato paste, thyme and bay leaf and cook for about 1 minute.
6. Stir in the broth and bring to a boil.

7. Reduce the heat to low and simmer, covered for about 1½ hours.

8. Stir in the mushrooms, celery, onion, carrot and garlic and simmers for about 40-60 minutes.

9. Stir in the salt and black pepper and remove from the heat.

10. Serve hot.

Nutrition: Calories: 447 Carbohydrates: 7.4g Protein: 30.8g Fat: 32.3g Sugar: 8g Sodium: 764mgFiber: 1.9g

CONCLUSION

The things to watch out for when coming off keto are weight gain, bloating, more energy, and feeling hungry. The weight gain is nothing to freak out over; perhaps, you might not even gain any. It all depends on your diet, how your body processes carbs, and, of course, water weight. The length of your keto diet is a significant factor in how much weight you have lost, which is caused by the reduction of carbs. The bloating will occur because of the reintroduction of fibrous foods and your body getting used to digesting them again. The bloating van lasts for a few days to a few weeks. You will feel like you have more energy because carbs break down into glucose, which is the body's primary source of fuel. You may also notice better brain function and the ability to work out more.

Whether you have met your weight loss goals, your life changes, or you simply want to eat whatever you want again. You cannot just suddenly start consuming carbs again for it will shock your system. Have an idea of what you want to allow back into your consumption slowly. Be familiar with portion sizes and stick to that amount of carbs for the first few times you eat post-keto.

Start with non-processed carbs like whole grain, beans, and fruits. Start slow and see how your body responds before resolving to add carbs one meal at a time.

The ketogenic diet is the ultimate tool you can use to plan your future. Can you picture being more involved, more productive and efficient, and more relaxed and energetic? That future is possible for you, and it does not have to be a complicated process to achieve that vision. You can choose right now to be healthier and slimmer and more fulfilled tomorrow. It is possible with the ketogenic diet.

It does not just improve your physical health but your mental and emotional health as well. This diet improves your health holistically. Do not give up now as there will be quite a few days where you may think to yourself, "Why am I doing this?" and to answer that, simply focus on the goals you wish to achieve.

A good diet enriched with all the proper nutrients is our best shot of achieving an active metabolism and efficient lifestyle. A lot of people think that the Keto diet is simply for people who are interested in losing weight. You will find that it is quite the opposite. There are intense keto diets where only 5 percent of the diet comes from carbs, 20 percent is from protein, and 75 percent is from fat. But even a modified version of this which involves consciously choosing foods low in carbohydrate and high in healthy fats is good enough.

Thanks for reading this book. I hope it has provided you with enough insight to get you going. Don't put off getting started. The sooner you begin this diet, the sooner you'll start to notice an improvement in your health and well-being.

CPSIA information can be obtained
at www.ICGtesting.com
Printed in the USA
BVHW011217080421
604483BV00009B/155